STRENGTHENING YOUR IMMUNE SYSTEM THROUGH DIET

Stay strong, generate low fat, live longer,easy ways to overcome illness through food

By

Barbara R. Latham

Strengthening your immune system through food

Copyright

Disclaimer

The information provided in the "NutriVitality" is for general informational purposes only. Although every attempt has been made to offer accurate and current information, the publisher and author disclaim all explicit and implied warranties and representations on the availability,correctness,appropriateness, completeness and reliability of the material embedded within.

The author and the publisher disclaim any liability of any loss or damage arising from reliance on the information provided in the NutriVitality.Readers are encouraged to consult with a healthcare professional or qualified nutritionist for individualized advice regarding their dietary choices.

Any reliance you place on the information in this cookbook NutriVitality is at your own risk. The author and the publisher will not be liable for any losses and damages in connection with the use of this cookbook.

Strengthening your
immune system through
food

About the Author

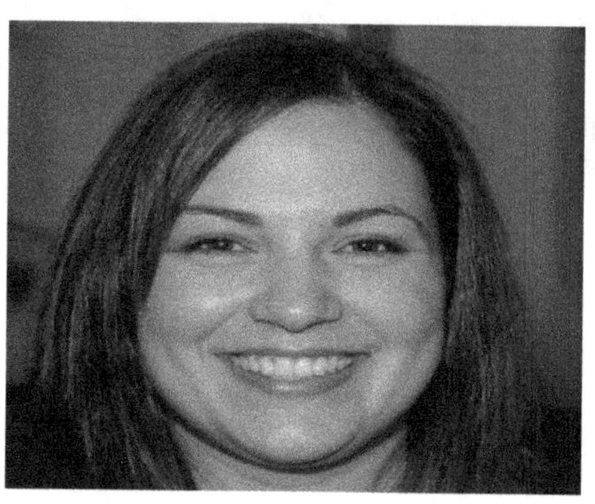

Hi there! I'm Barbara R. Latham, a chef who's incredibly passionate about discovering how food can be a powerful tool for healing our bodies. Cooking isn't just my profession; it's my way of exploring the incredible connection between what we eat and how our bodies respond to it.

Over the years, I've dedicated myself to mastering the art of creating delicious meals while also understanding the incredible impact food has on our well-being. My journey in the kitchen opened my eyes to something profound:

the immense potential of food to heal and strengthen our bodies from the inside out.

Driven by my love for food and a burning curiosity about its impact on health, I've delved into extensive research. I wanted to understand how the things we eat can truly boost our immune systems and contribute to our overall wellness.

In my book, I pour out all the knowledge I've gathered over the years. It's not just about recipes; it's a guide filled with tips and insights on how specific foods can truly bolster our immune systems. My goal is to share this understanding and inspire you to embrace a lifestyle where the foods you eat aren't just delicious but also work wonders in helping your body heal and thrive.

I believe in the incredible power of food to transform our health, and through my book, I

hope to empower you to make informed choices
that lead to a healthier and happier life. Cheers
to good food and good health!

Table of content

CHAPTER 1
CHAPTER 2
CHAPTER 3
CHAPTER 4
CHAPTER 5
CHAPTER 6
CHAPTER 7
CHAPTER 8
CHAPTER 9
CHAPTER 10

INTRODUCTION

Welcome to "NutriVitality: Unleashing Your
Body's Healing Power Through Food"!

In this book, we're diving into an amazing world where the food you eat isn't just about filling your stomach – it's about unlocking your body's incredible ability to heal itself. Imagine understanding how the things on your plate can become the key to feeling better, stronger, and healthier!

Throughout these pages, we'll explore how what you eat plays a massive role in not just your fitness but also in how your body fights off illnesses and repairs itself. It's not just a diet plan; it's a way to understand how food can literally help you become a healthier version of yourself.

Join me on this journey of discovery, where we'll reveal the secrets behind certain nutrients, the magic of different foods, and how they work together to keep you well. Let's learn together how your meals can be your allies in staying fit, strong, and full of vitality.

Strengthening your immune system through food

Strengthening your immune system through food

CHAPTER 1

IMMUNITY

Immunity refers to the body's ability to resist or fight off potential threats such as infections, diseases, or harmful substances. It involves a complex network of cells, tissues, and organs that work together to defend the body against invaders like viruses, bacteria, parasites, and other foreign substances.

There are two main types of immunity: innate immunity, which provides immediate but general defenses against a wide range of threats, and adaptive immunity, which develops more slowly and specifically targets particular invaders based on previous exposure or immunization. The immune system plays a crucial role in maintaining overall health by recognizing and neutralizing harmful agents while distinguishing them from the body's own healthy cells.

The immune system is an intricate defense mechanism that safeguards our body against various harmful elements that could cause illnesses or infections. It's akin to a vigilant army, comprising numerous specialized cells, tissues, organs, and chemical processes, all working harmoniously to protect us.

1. **Innate Immunity**:This is our body's first line of defense. It acts immediately upon encountering a threat, providing a general defense mechanism. Physical barriers like our skin, mucous membranes, and stomach acid, as well as certain cells like macrophages and neutrophils, form the frontline of innate immunity.

2. **Adaptive Immunity**:This is a more specialized form of defense that develops over time. It comes into play when the innate system isn't enough to combat a specific threat.

Adaptive immunity "learns" from past encounters; it remembers specific pathogens and its infections.

Strengthening your immune system through food

CHAPTER 2

ACTIVATE YOUR IMMUNE COMMAND CENTER

Supporting your safe framework includes sustaining your body in different ways.

First and foremost, we should discuss food. Eating a wide assortment of organic products, veggies, entire grains, lean proteins (like poultry, fish, beans), and sound fats (tracked down in nuts, avocados, and olive oil) resembles providing your resistant framework with an increase in superpowers. These food varieties are loaded with fundamental supplements, nutrients, and cell reinforcements that assist your body with working at its ideal.

In any case, it's not just about what's on your plate; development matters as well! Getting your body rolling through work out, whether it's an energetic walk, yoga, or moving to your number one tunes, can fortify your invulnerable framework. It resembles giving your body a well disposed bump to remain honest and be prepared to shield itself.

Rest is one more unrecognized yet truly great individual in the resistance domain. At the point when you get those Z's, your body goes into fix mode, fixing and restoring itself. It resembles raising a ruckus around town button and allowing your resistant framework to re-energize for the day ahead.

Furthermore, hello, stress is a tricky easily overlooked detail that can play with your insusceptible framework. Tracking down ways of unwinding — whether it's through contemplation, side interests, or essentially resting — can do ponders for your insusceptibility. It resembles offering your body

a reprieve, allowing it to zero in on keeping you
solid as opposed to worrying.

Remaining hydrated is likewise critical!
Consider water your body's closest companion,
helping flush out poisons and keeping
everything chugging along as expected.

Strengthening your immune system through food

CHAPTER 3

STARVE YOUR DISEASE FEED YOUR HEALTH

"Starve Your Infection, Feed Your Wellbeing" resembles a mantra for supporting your body to battle sicknesses and advance generally health.

Picture this: Envision your body as a nursery. Similarly as you'd water the plants you need to flourish and eliminate the weeds that obstruct their development, a similar guideline applies to your wellbeing.

At the point when we say "starve your infection," it implies denying those components that could hurt your prosperity. This incorporates avoiding handled food sources, over the top sugars, undesirable fats, and fake added substances. These resemble the weeds that can gag the essentialness out of your body, encouraging a climate where illnesses could flourish.

Presently, "feed your well being" is tied in with giving your body the supplements it necessities to thrive. Settle on entire, supplement thick food sources overflowing with nutrients, minerals, and cell reinforcements. Organic products, vegetables, lean proteins, sound fats — these are the sustaining components that carry on like daylight and water, supporting your body's strength and imperativeness.

It resembles allowing your body the most ideal opportunity to flourish by picking food sources that help its regular protections and generally prosperity. Keep in mind, little changes in what you eat can have an immense effect by they way you feel and how your body wards off sicknesses. Thus, by "starving your sickness"

Strengthening your
immune system through
food

and "taking care of your wellbeing," you're
basically developing a better, more joyful you
from the back to front.

Strengthening your immune system through food

CHAPTER 4

REGENERATES YOUR HEALTH

4 Strategies to regenerate your body and feel youthful

Our bodies are continually modifying ourselves, and that implies we as a whole get the opportunity to further develop our bodies extraordinarily and, likewise, our wellbeing — beginning at this point. This is the way to tackle the force of recovery. For reasons unknown, your body has different recovery modes. We'll call the less supportive one the 'slow technician' and the ideal one the 'youthful specialist'. You can pick which body fix technician will accomplish the work, specialists currently accept. The key? Work out

Recollect that your hereditary coding did not depend on life as it is lived today, however as it was lived a long time prior.

"Without active work, your body infers that it is winter — in a real sense"

On the off chance that you were lounging around many days back, it ordinarily implied it was the chilly climate season, with you and your family clustered together inside for warmth, long past the season for social affair and hunting. Also, that implied that your body expected to move into hibernation mode; as a matter of fact, your main concern is consume as not many kilojoules as could really be expected. So the sluggish repairman dominated, accomplishing negligible work and permitting your unresolved issues, your muscles to debilitate and that's only the tip of the iceberg. Yet, assuming that you get up and move around each day, your hereditary coding says, 'Aha! I really want more grounded bones and muscles, more synapses to resolve how to chase that wild hog and a more grounded cardiovascular framework to keep everything provided with oxygen and supplements while I scrounge for nuts and berries in the forest'. Then, the youthful specialist will work, reinforcing key body frameworks and making solid, new cells. There are four methodologies that have shown to be awesome for supporting your body's maintenance framework and guarantee that the youthful repairman is accomplishing the work.

Strategy one: Exercise

The new Wellspring of Youth: an everyday stroll in addition to three strength-instructional meetings every week. As referenced, energizing examination is demonstrating that actual work flips the adolescent switch, motioning toward your body to become more youthful as it fixes, keeps up with and recovers itself. Among the key body frameworks that advantage:

Muscles

In one exploration study, 70-year-olds who embraced ordinary strength-preparing exercise were all around as solid as 28-year-olds who didn't work out. In the event that you skip work out, you'll lose muscle strength as time passes.

Mind

Once, specialists accepted that age-related drops in memory and mental abilities were the unavoidable aftereffect of kicking the bucket synapses. Presently, researchers realize that the cerebrum can fortify old cells and create new ones. Practice delivers a compost-like substance called BDNF.

Heart

A heart-threatening lifestyle—replete with high-fat foods, too many kilojoules, little exercise, and smoking—can leave you with stiff, clogged arteries 40 years older than your biological age.

Aging also weakens the heart's ability to contract and pump blood. Exercise makes heart muscle contract more forcefully, makes arteries more supple and slows atherosclerosis.

Bones

Your skeleton grows lighter with time. But research shows that strength-training pumps up the body's natural bone-building system so that bone density increases.
Without it, you can lose 2 percent of your bone density per year, raising your risk of fractures.

Strategy two: Shed stress, make connections

Individuals' minds are designed for life in gatherings. All things considered, in ancient times the most secure spot to be was in a gathering. So when we're disconnected, our feelings of anxiety ascend; to our psyche minds, delayed times of confinement aren't protected or normal, so our cerebrums answer by delivering pressure synthetics to urge us right into it.

Some evidence of the strong impact that pressure decrease and social associations can have on your body's maintenance framework:

- Men who endure a coronary failure are multiple times less inclined to kick the bucket from a subsequent respiratory failure in the event that they get back home to relatives than if they return to a vacant home

- Women with additional companions and family members in their lives are bound to endure coronary illness and disease than those with few

- People with coronary illness who had been restless, however at that point brought down their feelings of anxiety, essentially cut their gamble of a cardiovascular failure

Strategy three: Supply the correct 'parts

A new car won't run with replacement engine parts pulled from a beaten-up car. And your body won't be able to repair itself with the wrong parts, either. Every time you eat junk food, refined sugars or grain products such as white bread, trans fat and highly processed foods, you're doing just that.

Nature's top-of-the-line parts list for the human body are all the nutrients you'll find in lean protein, oily fish, nuts, berries and—especially—antioxidant-rich fruit and vegetables.

The proof that it works:

- Every everyday serving of veggies you add to your eating regimen cuts your coronary illness risk by 4% (or more) and your stroke risk by 3 to 5 percent

- Just five servings of products of the soil a day lower diabetes risk by 39%

- Subjects matured 70 and more established who ate the freshest produce, in one Australian review, had the least kinks

- Eating an additional one apple daily could decrease your gamble of an early passing by 20% — this was the decision of a UK concentrate on that deliberate blood levels of L-ascorbic acid (a marker of organic product utilization) in very nearly 20,000 individuals. Adding at least two day to day divides of products of the soil could generally split your gamble, paying little mind to mature, pulse or smoking propensities

Strategy four: Ditch the stuff that interferes with repair

Smoking. Exposure to second-hand smoke. Drinking to excess. This bad stuff thwarts your body's regeneration efforts. The upside—study after study proves that your body's repair system goes back to work the moment you give them up:

- Not long after halting smoking, your lungs and cardiovascular framework start fixing themselves. Pulse falls more like a better level in 8 hours or less. In somewhere around 24 hours, your coronary episode risk starts to fall. In no less than a month, lungs work better

- Your mind can fix itself even after harm caused by weighty drinking. In a US review from the College of California, San Francisco, scientists found that heavy drinkers who remained sober for almost seven years proceeded as well as non-drunkards in mind capability tests

- Respiratory failure rates among non-smokers plunged while a smoking boycott was founded in cafés and bars in a single medium-sized American town — something scientists property to a drop in openness to recycled smoke

Strengthening your immune system through food

CHAPTER 5

FEED YOUR INNER ECOSYSTEM

Have you at any point viewed that you are a
delightful indication of nature?
That the very knowledge that you find in the
regular world is the insight that made you?
We are presently seeing the fine difficult
exercise that should be regarded for our planet's
environment to work ideally and to help life.
We also have a fragile environment that can
prosper with the right fixings.
Caring for ourselves is so significant on the
grounds that it makes us more grounded and
more powerful with regards to rewarding others,
and to nature.

• Move

Your body loves to move, it is intended to move.
Permit development to feel like a joy and not a
task. Take part in classes that rouse you (not
worry you) and move outside at whatever point
you can, a day to day walk or a dip in the sea can

completely reset your outlook and a portion of vitamin D does ponder.

• Rest

The human heart rests two times however much it thumps. What a brilliant plan. We are not intended to be in never-ending harvest and efficiency. Rest is similarly pretty much as significant as action. Useful rest and adequate rest permit your brain and body to process and to recuperate profoundly

• Drink

The human grown-up body is composed of around 60-70% water. Water transports supplements to your cells, it hydrates your mind which will work on mental lucidity and focus and supports the sound working of your inward organs. The best measure of water to be polished off every day is 2.5 - 3.5 liters.

Here are some of water hacks:

- Begin the day with an enormous cup of warm water and new lemon (which will assist with hydrating you and to help your stomach related framework)
- Buy a reusable glass bottle that you can fill and drink two times a day
- Add Doterra natural oils or new organic products/spices to your water to captivate you to drink more regularly.
- **Breathe**

We inhale 20,000 times each day - on the off chance that you can further develop something that you do this frequently it will, presumably, immensely affect your life. Pause for a minute, notice your breath. Take in and out through your nose. Take in for 3 seconds and out for 3 seconds. Permit your tummy to ascend as you breathe in and to fall as you breathe out.

At the point when your breath is quiet your sensory system realizes that it is protected and it can focus on recuperating (which isn't vital when you are in endurance mode). At the point when your breath is quiet your psyche is quiet and it encounters an entirely different viewpoint of the real world.

• **Think**

We think on normal 60,000 considerations each day. That is 3 fold the number of contemplations as the breaths that we take each day! At the point when we have a thought, our body has a quick physiological reaction. Contemplate an upsetting situation and you can in a real sense produce more cortisol and adrenaline, envision a blissful idea, your muscles unwind and you can create more oxytocin and serotonin.

What considerations would you say you are thinking? Could it be said that they are moving you toward your longings and the sentiments that you might want to feel?

"The fastest way to change your body is to change your mind" – Eric Franklin.

• **Joy**

Encircle yourself with individuals, books, places, web recordings and anything that encourages you. At the point when you feel great your entire framework will respond, your pressure delivers, your resistant framework is supported, you inhale all the more completely and you connect diversely with your general surroundings.

• **Listen**

However insane as it might sound - your body seems to be continuously conversing with you. Your cerebrum and body are organizations of correspondence which work constantly to keep a feeling of harmony in your body and psyche.

By requiring a moment, seeing your breath, paying attention to your pulse, detecting the strain you might be holding, you can dial into this steady correspondence and work with it. Your body will just talk stronger until you start to hear it (neck pressure, spinal pain, tension) and when you in all actuality do tune in and make a move on it's solicitations it will be so thankful and all things considered, diseases will die down.

• Eat

The stomach microbiome has 60-80% of the body's safe cells and an expected 90% of the serotonin that you produce (the key chemical that settles our state of mind, sensations of prosperity, and joy) is delivered in the stomach.

Support your stomach with as many plant based food sources as you can to work on the variety of it's microbiome, eat matured food sources and refreshments (fermented tea, sauerkraut) or more all partake in your food, 'make a dinner of it' permit yourself an opportunity to process the staggering fuel that you are devouring.

• Nature

Being in nature amazingly affects our psychological and actual prosperity, lessening circulatory strain, pulse, muscle pressure, and the creation of stress chemicals.

Is it conceivable to roll out little improvements to your way of life so you can procure the beneficial outcomes of being in nature somewhat more? Have your morning meal outside toward the beginning of the day? Develop your own veggies? Set out on an everyday walk? Wrap up warm and get outside to partake in the nightfall?

Strengthening your immune system through food

CHAPTER 6

THE 5 × 5 × 5 FRAMEWORK : EATING TO BEAT DISEASE

The "5 × 5 × 5 Structure: Eating to Beat Sickness" is like a guide directing you toward better well being through food decisions. Envision it as a tool stash loaded with systems to engage your body in its battle against illnesses.

- **5 Principles**: These are the core values that shape your dietary patterns. They include components like assortment, balance, control, supplement thickness, and care. For example, consider having a rainbow of products of the soil on your plate (assortment), offsetting your dinners with the right extents of proteins, sugars, and fats (balance), not exaggerating any one nutrition type (control), picking food varieties wealthy in supplements (supplement thickness), and being aware of what and how you eat (care).

- **5 Food Groups**:These address the vital classes of food sources that you ought to integrate into your eating routine. It incorporates organic products, vegetables, entire grains, lean proteins, and sound fats. For instance, natural products like berries loaded with cell reinforcements, veggies, for example, mixed greens loaded up with nutrients, entire grains like quinoa or earthy colored rice for fiber, lean proteins like chicken or tofu, and sound fats like avocados or nuts.

- **5 Benefits**: This part underscores the prizes of following this system. It prompts further developed insusceptibility, better energy levels, decreased aggravation, upgraded processing, and generally speaking prosperity. Envision feeling more vigorous over the course of the day, encountering less throbbing painfulness, having a more grounded insusceptible framework to ward off diseases, and simply feeling better from within.

The enchantment of this structure lies in its effortlessness and flexibility. There's really no need to focus on severe eating regimens or hardship; it's tied in with settling on careful decisions inside these boundaries to help your body's inherent capacity to remain solid and fend off illnesses. By embracing this structure, you're basically furnishing your body with the devices it requires to flourish and safeguard itself against different medical problems.

Strengthening your immune system through food

CHAPTER 7

RETHINKING THE KITCHEN

"Reevaluating the Kitchen" with the "5 × 5 × 5 System: Eating to Beat Infection" resembles giving your kitchen a total makeover, however rather than new cupboards or ledges, you're loading it with the structure blocks for better wellbeing.

Picture your kitchen as a center of wellbeing, where every fixing is painstakingly decided to squeeze into this system:

- **Embracing the Principles**: It's tied in with making little yet effective changes. Take a stab at adding beautiful veggies to your shopping list every week, guaranteeing an equilibrium of supplements in your feasts, keeping away from limits in any one nutrition class, and enjoying each nibble with care.

- **Diversifying the Food Groups**:Change your refrigerator and storage room into gold mines of wellbeing! Load up on new natural products, energetic veggies, entire grains, lean proteins like chicken or beans, and sound fats like avocados or olive oil.

- **Reaping the Benefits**:This kitchen upset isn't just about delicious dinners; it's tied in with feeling improved as well! Envision having more energy to handle your day, feeling more grounded and better inside, and giving your body the apparatuses it necessitates to avert sicknesses.

By reexamining your kitchen and adjusting it to the "5 × 5 × 5 System," you're basically transforming it into a force to be reckoned with for advancing your prosperity. It's not necessary to focus on exceptional changes but instead about supporting your body with the right

fixings to help it flourish and remain versatile
against wellbeing challenges.

Rethinking Your Kitchen

It may be time to rethink your kitchen. Do you
have the core essentials you need to cook
healthy meals? Are your cooking implements
healthy to use? Or are you cooking using plastic
utensils and Teflon-coated pans? Step one is to
audit your kitchen. Here are a few things to
have on hand in the kitchen:

- A high-quality knife set
- A metal colander
- At least one (1) high quality pan (cast
  iron, stainless steel or ceramic non-stick –
  NOT TEFLON)
- Vegetable peeler
- Wooden spoon
- Glass storage containers

Things to throw out:

- Plastic Tupperware containers. Use glass / pyrex. Plastic lids are OK, but NEVER microwave them.
- Plastic water bottles. Use metal or glass instead.

Things to stock in your pantry:

- Extra virgin olive oil
- Balsamic vinegar
- Spices
- Whole grains
- Wild Rice
- Whole wheat pasta
- Coffee
- Tea
- Tree nuts
- Tinned seafood
- Sauces

Long-term keepers (years):

- Peppercorns
- Tea
- Pasta

Months:

- Dried beans 9 months
- Spices 6 months

Strengthening your
immune system through
food

CHAPTER 8

EXCEPTIONAL FOODS

I've generally adopted a characteristic food-based strategy, and a lot of my eating regimen is motivated by a remarkable mix of two of the best food societies in the reality where individuals age better and are by and large better.

The following are six staples eating that can assist you with helping insusceptible wellbeing and remain sound:

1. Fruits

Apples: An apple daily could ward the specialist off, however three apples daily can assist with decreasing muscle to fat ratio. They're flexible, extraordinary for servings of mixed greens, and delectable as a bite or heated in a sweet.

Pears: Pears are a great wellspring of dietary fiber (a medium-sized organic product has 6 grams) for stomach wellbeing.

Pro tip: to track down a ready pear, hold the natural product by its base with one hand, and with the other, squeeze the tissue at the lower part of the stem. On the off chance that the tissue gives somewhat, it's prepared to eat.

Grapefruit: Grapefruit tissue contains illness battling flavonoids and L-ascorbic acid, which is a strong DNA-safeguarding cell reinforcement and mitigating substance.

Avocados: The fats in avocados are solid monounsaturated unsaturated fats, which can decrease blood levels of awful LDL cholesterol and bring down your gamble of coronary illness.

2. **Vegetables**

Broccoli: Broccoli is strong in sulforaphane, which safeguards foundational microorganisms, further develops stomach wellbeing and digestion, and enhances resistant reactions.

Soy: Soy is eaten as a bean, made into tofu, matured, and could in fact be changed into wine. It has been related to bringing down the gamble of cardiovascular illness by 20% and diabetes by 23%.

Carrots: An old root vegetable that started in Southwest Asia, carrots are a decent wellspring of dietary fiber for stomach wellbeing. A half cup of ground carrot has 2 grams of fiber.

Mushrooms: Mushrooms contain a solvent fiber called beta-D-glucan, which invigorates guards to develop fresh blood vessels required for mending wounds. Simultaneously, it can keep destructive veins from taking care of tumors.

3. Legumes

White beans: Beans are a nutritious food that can assist with lessening cardiovascular gamble factors by bringing down blood cholesterol levels. They additionally contain important supplements like iron, zinc, magnesium and folate.

Lentils: Lentils are an exemplary vegetable in Mediterranean food. A half cup of dry lentils contains 18 grams of fiber, which is the greater part of the suggested day to day consumption for people.

4. **Bottles and jars**

Extra virgin olive oil (EVOO): EVOO is the best type of olive oil. The "additional virgin" alludes to oil that isn't refined, and thus, contains smidgens of ready olives. The oil and pieces are the wellspring of strong polyphenols that actuate wellbeing protections.

At the point when I purchase EVOO, I filter the mark on the container to distinguish which olive varieties were utilized. Many are produced using different olives, which can taste exceptionally pleasant, yet I favor monovarietal oil, which is less inclined to be weakened with less expensive oils.

Apple cider vinegar: Investigations have discovered that the acidic corrosive in apple juice vinegar decreases muscle to fat ratio, further develops insulin awareness, and brings down glucose.

Fermented bean paste: Walk around the center passageways of any Asian supermarket, and you'll see numerous sorts of matured bean glue. Produced using aged soy, they contain bioactives that battle fat cells.

5. Seafood

Salmon: Salmon is high in omega-3s, which get assimilated into fat cells and are utilized. Then, at that point, they make proteins that are delivered like cell firemen into the encompassing fat mass to stifle the irritation brought about by fat.

Roe: Assuming you're investigating extraordinary preferences, you should attempt the roe (eggs) of specific shellfishes. Roe is normally loaded with omega-3s, so it takes surprisingly little to get a significant portion of sound fats.

Sardine: Sardines are a respected fish of the Mediterranean. They contain bioactives that can further develop digestion and lower blood cholesterol.

6. Liquids

Matcha tea: Matcha is a green tea known for its clear green tone. Investigations have discovered that matcha can counter the metabolic impacts of a high-fat eating regimen.

Oolong tea: A concentrate by the U.S. Branch of Horticulture showed that drinking six cups of oolong tea three days seven days worked on by and large digestion.

Strengthening your
immune system through
food

CHAPTER 9

SAMPLE MEAL GUIDE AND RECIPES

- ### HEALTHY CHOCOLATE MOUSSE

Serves 4

Prep time: 5 minutes

Cooking time: 5 minutes + 30 minutes set time

Ingredients

4 ounces dark chocolate (70% cacao or greater), chopped into 1-inch pieces 12 ounces silken tofu

2 tablespoons maple syrup

Chopped tree nuts (walnuts, hazelnuts, pecans), for garnish Blueberries, strawberries, and /or blackberries, for garnish Fresh mint or lavender, for garnish (optional)

Preparation

• In a double boiler, melt the chocolate over medium heat, stirring periodically to prevent scorching. When the chocolate has completely melted, add the silken tofu and maple syrup.

Stir to combine.

• Transfer the mixture to a food processor and whip until fluffy.

• Spoon the mousse into individual ramekins or serving cups. Place in the refrigerator to cool and set for at least 30 minutes.

• To serve, garnish with crushed nuts, berries, and mint leaves

• CAULIFLOWER COUSCOUS with KALE and CABBAGE

Makes 4 servings

Preparation time: 15 minutes

Cooking time: 0 minutes

Ingredients

½ head cauliflower, grated (4 cups)| 2 cups red cabbage, thinly sliced

2 cups tightly packed dino kale, thinly sliced*

5 stalks green onion, chopped (3/4 cup)

1 cup dried cranberries

I cup raw walnuts, chopped 2 tablespoons olive oil

¼ cup fresh lemon juice

2 tablespoons stone ground mustard

Salt and cracked pepper to taste

Preparation

• Rinse all of the vegetables very well and pat dry.

• Remove the stems on the cauliflower, chop the head in half, and grate one of the halves using a box grater (note: you can also pulse cauliflower florets in a food processor).

• Add cauliflower couscous, cabbage, kale, green onion, dried cranberries, and walnuts to a large serving bowl.

• Whisk together the olive oil, lemon juice, and stone ground mustard together in a small bowl. Pour it over the veggies and toss everything together well.

• **ROASTED BRANZINO**

Servings: 4 servings

Cooking Time: 15 minutes

Prep Time: 30 minutes

Ingredients

2 whole branzino, scaled and gutted

2 Belgian endives, thinly sliced

1 leek, thinly sliced

1 cup cherry tomatoes, halved

4 cloves garlic, thinly sliced

4 sprigs rosemary

2 tbsp fresh parsley, chopped

1 lemon, sliced into rounds

4 tbsp extra virgin olive oil

Fine sea salt

Black pepper

Preparation

• Preheat oven to 425°F

• Rinse fish and make cuts down the sides.

Stuff each fish with 2 rosemary sprigs and 2 lemon slices. Combine 3 tablespoons of the olive oil and the parsley, and rub over the outside of the fish.

• Toss the Belgian endives and leeks in the remaining 1 tablespoon of olive oil, tomatoes, and garlic slices, and season with salt and pepper.

• Line a baking sheet with parchment, and spread the vegetables over in a thin la Top with fish.

• Bake for 20-30 minutes, until the fish is cooked through and the vegetables are tender.

- **MEDITERRANEAN VEGETABLE SPAGHETTI**

Makes 2 servings

Preparation time: 15 minutes

Cooking time: 20 minutes

Ingredients

1 red pepper, diced

1 yellow pepper, diced

2 plum tomatoes, sliced into eighths

A dozen cherry tomatoes

1 zucchini/courgette

1 bowl of spinach

Λ handful of black olives

2 tbsp of tomato puree

½ a jalapeño pepper (optional)

2 tbsp of dried herbs de provence

2 tbsp of apple cider vinegar or the juice of 1
lime salt

1 box whole wheat spaghetti

Preparation

• Put the pasta water over high heat and bring to
a boil. Add the pasta and cook according to
package instructions.

• Heat olive oil in a saute pan over medium high heat, and add the chopped peppers, plum tomatoes, and herbs de provence.

• Allow the mix to simmer and gently disintegrate to form the sauce. After a few minutes add the tomato puree and the apple cider vinegar or lime juice.

• Slice the zucchini in half before chopping it into thin half moon shapes, place these to one side as you cut the cherry tomatoes into quarters.

• Once the vegetables in the sauce mixture begin to break down, add the cherry tomatoes, zucchini slices, and spinach, mixing them in well to cook for about 5-7 minutes.

• Drain the pasta and stir it into the sauce. Stir in the olives, and top with additional herbs.

Strengthening your
immune system through
food

CHAPTER 10

TWENTY - FIVE IMMUNE -BOOSTING

Boosting your immune system through food is essential for overall health. Here are 25 immune-boosting foods that can support your body's defenses:

1. Citrus fruits (e.g., oranges, lemons, grapefruits) rich in vitamin C.

2. Berries (e.g., strawberries, blueberries, raspberries) packed with antioxidants.

3. Leafy greens (e.g., spinach, kale) filled with vitamins and minerals.

4. Garlic, known for its antimicrobial properties.

5. Ginger, known for its anti-inflammatory and antioxidant effects.

6. Turmeric, containing curcumin with potent anti-inflammatory properties.

7. Yogurt or kefir with probiotics for gut health.

8. Almonds, providing vitamin E and healthy fats.

9. Sunflower seeds, high in phosphorus, magnesium, and vitamin E.

10. Green tea, rich in antioxidants like catechins.

11. Papaya, loaded with vitamins C, A, and folate.

12. Kiwi, abundant in vitamin C, K, and antioxidants.

13. Poultry (e.g., chicken, turkey) for zinc and high-quality protein.

14. Shellfish (e.g., oysters, crab) rich in zinc and selenium.

15. Bell peppers, particularly red ones, high in vitamin C.

16. Broccoli, offering vitamins A, C, and E, as well as antioxidants.

17. Carrots, abundant in beta-carotene, are converted into vitamin A.

18. Sweet potatoes, packed with beta-carotene, fiber, and vitamins.

19. Mushrooms containing beta-glucans for immune support.

20. Salmon and other fatty fish with omega-3 fatty acids.

21. Tuna, providing vitamin D and omega-3s.

22. Seeds (e.g., chia seeds, flaxseeds) loaded with nutrients and fiber.

23. Legumes (e.g., lentils, chickpeas) for plant-based protein and fiber.

24. Dark chocolate (in moderation), rich in antioxidants like flavonoids.

25. Fermented foods (e.g., kimchi, sauerkraut)
for gut health and immunity.

Incorporating these immune-boosting foods into
your diet can contribute to a stronger immune
system, aiding your body's ability to fight off
illnesses and maintain overall well-being.

CONCLUSION

In conclusion, the book delves deep into the fascinating world of enhancing your immune system through the power of food. Throughout its pages, it has unraveled a treasure trove of information about 25 incredible immune-boosting foods, each serving as a key to fortify your body's defenses.

By exploring these foods, their nutrients, and their remarkable benefits, the book aims to empower you with the knowledge needed to make informed choices about your diet. It's not just about what you eat but how these foods can be your allies in supporting a resilient immune system and overall health.

Remember, incorporating these immune-boosting foods into your meals isn't just a one-time action; it's a lifestyle choice. It's about embracing a diverse array of nutrient-rich foods that can nourish and protect your body every day.

As you journey through the content, may you find inspiration and practical guidance to transform your eating habits and, ultimately, bolster your body's ability to ward off illnesses and thrive. Here's to a healthier, immune-strong you!

Review page
Dear Reader,

I hope this message finds you well. I wanted to take a moment to express my gratitude for your support and for choosing to explore my book. Your interest in NutriVitality means a lot to me.

I'd greatly appreciate it if you could spare a few moments to share your thoughts and feelings about the book. Your feedback is incredibly valuable and helps me understand how the content resonated with you. Whether it's a few sentences or a detailed review, your insights will

provide invaluable guidance for me and for
potential readers.

Your review could help others considering this
book to make an informed decision, and it would
mean the world to me to hear your thoughts on
your reading experience.

Thank you so much for your time and
consideration. Your feedback truly matters.

Warm regards,
Barbara R. Latham